Lose weight without diets and drugs (easy, healthy, simple)

Introduction

- The importance of proper nutrition for health and weight loss

- Why juices and smoothies help effectively lose weight

- Benefits of using juices and smoothies: vitamin saturation, metabolism support, ease of preparation

- Greens and spices: parsley, cilantro, ginger, turmeric, cinnamon

- Superfoods and supplements: spirulina, chia, flax seeds, maca, matcha

- How to combine foods for maximum benefit

Chapter 3: Diet and nutrition plan

page -38

- Sample weekly and monthly diet to achieve results

- How to properly incorporate juices and smoothies into your daily diet without giving up other foods

- Tips for creating a balanced diet based on your daily calorie intake

- Sample meal plans with juices and smoothies:

- Detox program

- Accelerated weight loss plan (7 days)

- Examples of a diet for keeping weight with the inclusion of juices and smoothies

- How to adapt drinks depending on the season and personal preferences

Conclusion

- Summary: Health and slimness through proper nutrition

- Motivation and inspiration for supporting a new lifestyle

- A reminder of the benefits and simplicity of juices and smoothies in achieving and keeping weight

Introduction

The Power of Smoothies and Juices for Health and Weight Loss

In our fast-paced world, prioritizing health can feel challenging. Many people struggle to find the time, energy, and resources to support a balanced diet, let alone one that promotes weight loss and sustained energy. Smoothies and juices offer a convenient, nutrient-packed solution to these common obstacles, serving as powerful allies in weight management and overall wellness. These beverages are simple to prepare, easily customizable, and incredibly versatile, making them an excellent fit for those seeking a healthier lifestyle without excessive effort.

Why Smoothies and Juices Work for Weight Loss

Weight loss is often associated with strict diets and restrictive eating, but smoothies and juices offer a gentler, more flexible approach. They can be integrated into any lifestyle and adjusted according to specific dietary needs or preferences. Unlike traditional weight-loss methods, which may demand calorie counting or complex meal planning, smoothies and juices offer a straightforward way to cut calories, improve nutrition, and enjoy a variety of flavors.

One of the primary reasons smoothies and juices support weight loss is their high nutrient density. Both options allow you to consume large amounts of vitamins, minerals, fiber, and antioxidants without the bulk or calories found in solid foods. These beverages can also be strategically crafted to help control appetite and promote satiety, which is essential for reducing overall caloric intake and curbing unhealthy cravings.

Moreover, incorporating a variety of nutrient-dense ingredients — such as leafy greens, low-sugar fruits, and protein-rich additions —

supports the body's metabolism and energy levels, allowing for more effective calorie burning throughout the day. Certain ingredients, like spinach, berries, ginger, and chia seeds, are particularly known for their metabolism-boosting properties, making them ideal for weight management.

The Health Benefits of Smoothies and Juices Beyond Weight Loss

While weight loss is a common goal, smoothies and juices offer a wide range of health benefits that extend far beyond slimming down. These beverages can serve as powerful tools for boosting immunity, improving digestion, enhancing energy levels, and supporting mental clarity. The high concentration of vitamins and antioxidants found in smoothies and juices helps the body combat oxidative stress, fight inflammation, and protect against illness.

Immune Support

Smoothies and juices made with ingredients like citrus fruits, ginger, and leafy greens can significantly enhance immune function. For example, vitamin C, found in citrus fruits and bell peppers, is a known immune booster that helps the body fight off colds and infections. Ingredients like turmeric and ginger have anti-inflammatory properties that can further strengthen the immune system.

Improved Digestion

Juices and smoothies are rich in dietary fiber, which aids digestion and promotes gut health. Smoothies keep all of the fiber from fruits and vegetables, which helps support regular bowel movements and prevents constipation. Fiber also feeds the beneficial bacteria in the gut, contributing to a healthier digestive system.

Enhanced Energy and Focus

Unlike sugary snacks or caffeine, which offer only temporary boosts, smoothies and juices provide sustained energy without sudden spikes and crashes. Ingredients like spinach, kale, and berries supply natural sources of energy and are high in antioxidants that support cognitive function. The slow release of nutrients from fiber-rich ingredients also helps support stable blood sugar levels, which can improve concentration and mental clarity.

Variety and Flexibility in a Balanced Diet

One of the greatest advantages of incorporating smoothies and juices into a diet is the variety and flexibility they offer. With countless combinations of fruits, vegetables, greens, nuts, seeds, and superfoods, these beverages can be tailored to suit almost any dietary preference or nutritional goal. Whether you're looking for a protein-packed breakfast smoothie, a refreshing green juice, or a post-workout recovery drink, there is a recipe to meet your needs.

Smoothies and juices also make it easier to enjoy nutrient-rich foods that you might not typically include in your diet. For instance, some people may find it challenging to eat enough leafy greens or certain vegetables in their regular meals. However, blending them into a smoothie with a handful of berries or a splash of almond milk can create a delicious and nutrient-dense drink. Similarly, juicing can help you incorporate ingredients like beets, ginger, and celery, which are rich in vitamins and minerals but may be less palatable on their own.

This flexibility allows for a gradual, sustainable approach to dietary changes. By adding one or two smoothies or juices a day, individuals can start to shift their eating patterns in a way that feels manageable and enjoyable. Over time, these small changes can lead to more consistent healthy eating habits, supporting long-term weight management and overall health.

Key Ingredients and Their Impact on Weight Loss

Smoothies and juices are more than just blended fruits and vegetables; they're carefully crafted combinations of ingredients that work together to support the body's needs. Including ingredients known to promote weight loss can significantly enhance the effectiveness of these beverages. Here are a few examples:

Leafy Greens: Spinach, kale, and arugula are low in calories but packed with fiber and essential nutrients, helping to keep you full without adding bulk. Leafy greens also have chlorophyll, which can help detoxify the body and improve digestion.

Low-Sugar Fruits: Berries, green apples, and citrus fruits provide sweetness without spiking blood sugar levels. These fruits are also high in antioxidants, which help fight inflammation and support metabolic health.

Healthy Fats: Adding a small amount of healthy fat, such as avocado, chia seeds, or almond butter, can make a smoothie more filling and satisfying. Healthy fats also aid in the absorption of fat-soluble vitamins, ensuring that you get the most out of the nutrients in your drink.

Protein: Including a source of protein, such as Greek yogurt, protein powder, or hemp seeds, can help stabilize blood sugar levels and keep you feeling full longer. Protein is especially beneficial for those who want to use smoothies as a meal replacement.

Transitioning to a Healthy Lifestyle

For many, the journey to a healthier lifestyle can seem daunting, especially with busy schedules and the abundance of unhealthy food options. Smoothies and juices provide a convenient entry point to healthier eating habits, making it easier to avoid processed foods and reach for nutrient-dense alternatives. They're quick to prepare, easy to customize, and can be enjoyed on the go, making them ideal for anyone with a hectic lifestyle.

Incorporating smoothies and juices into your routine is not just about achieving a specific weight loss goal. It's a way to nourish your body, discover new flavors, and build a sustainable foundation for lasting health. By focusing on quality ingredients and experimenting with flavors, you can create a personalized approach to wellness that is both enjoyable and effective. Over time, the benefits will extend far beyond the scale, positively affecting energy levels, mood, and overall vitality.

As we explore further in this book, you'll find a variety of recipes, meal plans, and tips for maximizing the benefits of smoothies and juices. With the right strategies, you can transform these beverages into powerful tools for weight management and overall well-being. Embrace the journey and enjoy the process of discovering delicious ways to take control of your health.

Chapter 1: Basics of Juices and Smoothies for Weight Loss

This chapter will cover foundational information about using juices and smoothies as effective tools for weight loss. We'll explore the unique benefits of each, principles for creating weight-loss-friendly beverages, and essential ingredients to include in your recipes.

Section 1: Understanding the Differences Between Juices and Smoothies

1. What is Juicing?

- Juicing involves extracting the liquid from fruits and vegetables, separating it from the fiber-rich pulp.

- As a result, juices have concentrated amounts of vitamins, minerals, and phytochemicals but lack fiber.

2. What is Blending?

- Blending, or making smoothies, involves pureeing whole fruits and vegetables, including their fiber, into a thick, drinkable form.

- Smoothies are filling because they keep all parts of the plant, including the fiber that helps promote satiety and improve digestion.

3. Key Benefits of Juices

- Rapid Nutrient Absorption: Without fiber, nutrients in juices are quickly absorbed, delivering a fast boost of energy and nutrients.

- Supports Detoxification: Juice cleanses are often used to give the digestive system a break while still delivering essential nutrients.

- Hydration: High-water-content ingredients, like cucumber and celery, make juices excellent for hydration.

4. Key Benefits of Smoothies

- Fiber for Fullness: Fiber slows digestion, helping you feel full longer and reducing overeating.

- Blood Sugar Control: The fiber in smoothies helps slow sugar absorption, keeping blood sugar levels more stable.

- Customizable for Different Goals: Smoothies can easily include protein, healthy fats, and superfoods to meet a variety of health and fitness goals.

5. When to Choose a Juice vs. a Smoothie

   - Juices: Ideal for a quick nutrient boost, as a pre-workout energy shot, or during a cleanse for digestive rest.

   - Smoothies: Best for meal replacement, managing hunger, and post-workout recovery due to the fiber and nutrient density.

6. Sample Section: The Essential Differences

   - "Understanding the difference between juices and smoothies is essential for effective weight loss. While juices cut fiber, allowing for rapid nutrient absorption, smoothies keep fiber, making them more filling and beneficial for digestion. Both options offer unique benefits and can be tailored to specific weight-loss goals."

Section 2: Foundational Principles of Weight-Loss Beverages

1. Balancing Macronutrients and Micronutrients

- Macronutrients: Include proteins, fats, and carbohydrates. For weight loss, aim for smoothies that include balanced portions of all three macronutrients.

    - Proteins: Greek yogurt, protein powder, nuts.

    - Healthy Fats: Avocado, chia seeds, flaxseeds.

    - Low-Sugar Carbohydrates: Leafy greens, berries, vegetables.

    - Micronutrients: Vitamins and minerals from a variety of colorful fruits and vegetables.

2. Choosing Low-Sugar, Fiber-Rich Ingredients

   - Benefits of Low-Sugar Choices: Minimizes calorie intake, reduces blood sugar spikes, and helps control cravings.

   - Fiber-Rich Ingredients: Fiber aids digestion, keeps you full, and reduces the temptation to snack on unhealthy foods.

   - Tips for Reducing Sugar Content:

   - Choose lower-sugar fruits like berries and green apples.

   - Use vegetables as a base (like spinach or kale) instead of higher-sugar fruits.

   - Avoid fruit juices or sweetened plant-based milks as liquid bases.

3. Creating Satiating Smoothies and Juices

   - Adding Protein and Fat for Satiety: Including protein (e.g., plant-based or whey protein powder) and healthy fats (e.g., almond butter) makes smoothies more filling.

   - Balanced Macronutrient Ratios: Aim for about 40% vegetables, 30% protein, and 30% healthy fats in weight-loss smoothies.

4. Sample Weight-Loss Beverage Ratios

   - Juices: 70% vegetables, 20% low-sugar fruits, 10% herbs or spices for flavor.

   - Smoothies**: 50% vegetables, 20% low-sugar fruits, 20% protein, 10% healthy fats.

Section 3: Core Ingredients for Weight Loss

1. Vegetables

- Leafy Greens: Spinach, kale, arugula - high in nutrients and low in calories.

- Cucumber and Celery: High water content for hydration, low in calories.

- Carrot and Beet: Higher in natural sugars but rich in antioxidants.

2. Low-Sugar Fruits

- Berries: Blueberries, strawberries, blackberries - low in sugar, high in antioxidants.

- Green Apple: Adds sweetness and fiber without too much sugar.

- Citrus Fruits: Lemons, limes, and grapefruit - great for flavor, low-calorie, and metabolism-boosting.

3. Healthy Fats

- Avocado: Creamy texture, healthy monounsaturated fats for satiety.

   - Nuts and Seeds: Almonds, chia seeds, flaxseeds – provide fiber and omega-3 fatty acids.

   - Coconut Oil or MCT Oil: Medium-chain triglycerides that boost metabolism and provide lasting energy.

4. Protein Sources

   - Greek Yogurt: High in protein, adds creaminess and slight tang.

   - Protein Powders: Choose plant-based or whey for extra protein.

   - Nut Butters: Almond or peanut butter adds protein and healthy fats.

5. Superfoods

   - Chia Seeds: Rich in omega-3s, fiber, and protein, making smoothies more filling.

   - Flaxseeds: Great source of fiber and omega-3s, helps with digestion.

- Spirulina and Matcha: High in antioxidants, supports metabolism and energy.

6. Flavor Enhancers

- Herbs and Spices: Mint, basil, cinnamon, ginger, and turmeric add flavor and offer health benefits, such as anti-inflammatory properties.

- Natural Sweeteners: If needed, use honey, stevia, or a small piece of banana for sweetness.

Sample Recipes and Practical Tips

1. Green Detox Juice

- Ingredients: Cucumber, celery, green apple, lemon, spinach, ginger.

- Benefits: Cleansing, hydrating, and low-calorie – great for a morning reset.

2. Protein-Packed Berry Smoothie

- Ingredients: Greek yogurt, mixed berries, chia seeds, spinach, almond milk.

- Benefits: High in protein and fiber, supports muscle recovery and keeps you full.

3. Avocado-Ginger Metabolism Booster

- *Ingredients: Avocado, green apple, spinach, lime juice, ginger, matcha powder.

- Benefits: Healthy fats and metabolism-boosting ingredients, keep you satisfied for hours.

4. Practical Tips for Preparation and Storage

- Prepping Ingredients: Chop vegetables and fruits in advance to save time. Freeze portions for quick access.

- Storage Tips: Juices are best consumed fresh, but smoothies can be stored for up to 24 hours in the fridge. Use airtight containers to minimize nutrient loss.

- Freezing Smoothie Packs: Prepare smoothie packs by portioning out ingredients in freezer bags. When ready to use, blend with liquid.

Section Summary: Crafting Weight-Loss Juices and Smoothies

In this section, we explored the essential elements of creating juices and smoothies that support weight loss. The balance of macronutrients and micronutrients is key to making beverages that not only taste good but also fulfill nutritional needs and keep you feeling full. By focusing on low-sugar, fiber-rich ingredients and including healthy fats and proteins, you can create satisfying drinks that fit seamlessly into your weight-loss plan. Each ingredient has been chosen for its unique benefits, whether it's providing hydration, fiber, antioxidants, or boosting metabolism. With these principles and core ingredients in mind, you can start crafting customized smoothies and juices that will support your weight-loss journey in a healthy, enjoyable way.

This expanded version of Chapter 1 covers the basics of juices and smoothies for weight loss, providing a clear understanding of the differences, benefits, and core components of each. With a variety of practical tips, recipes, and foundational principles, this chapter offers a comprehensive guide to making smoothies and juices a powerful part of your weight-loss strategy.

Chapter 2: Nutrient-Packed Ingredients and Their Benefits

In this chapter, we'll take an in-depth look at the core ingredients that make juices and smoothies not only nutritious but also effective for weight loss. We'll focus on the specific vegetables, fruits, herbs, spices, and superfoods that promote weight loss by supporting digestion, stabilizing blood sugar, and boosting metabolism. Each section will include examples of nutrient-packed ingredients, their health benefits, and practical tips for incorporating them into your weight-loss beverages.

Section 1: Vegetables for Weight Loss

1. The Power of Leafy Greens

   - Spinach: High in fiber and low in calories, spinach is rich in vitamins A, C, K, and folate. It's a versatile base for smoothies and juices that provides a mild flavor and helps to fill you up without adding many calories.

   - Kale: Known as a superfood, kale is packed with antioxidants, vitamins A and C, calcium, and fiber. Its nutrient density supports metabolism and energy levels, and it blends well with other ingredients for a rich, slightly earthy flavor.

   - Swiss Chard: This leafy green is a powerhouse of nutrients, including vitamin K, magnesium, and iron, which are essential for bone health and energy production.

2. Hydrating and Cleansing Vegetables

   - Cucumber: With its high-water content, cucumber is refreshing and hydrating, making it an excellent addition to any juice. It's also low in calories and helps flush out toxins, supporting a healthy digestive system.

   - Celery: Known for its diuretic properties, celery helps reduce water retention and bloating. It's low in calories and packed with antioxidants and fiber, aiding digestion and providing a subtle flavor that pairs well with other ingredients.

3. Roots for Digestive Health and Energy

   -Carrots: Rich in beta-carotene, carrots are excellent for skin health and immune support. They add natural sweetness and are a great source of fiber, which aids in digestion and keeps you feeling full.

- Beets: Beets are high in iron, fiber, and nitrates, which boost blood flow and support endurance. While they have natural sugars, they're low-calorie and provide a rich flavor when blended with other fruits and vegetables.

4. Cruciferous Vegetables for Metabolism Support

- Broccoli: Known for its metabolism-boosting and detoxifying effects, broccoli has high amounts of fiber, vitamin C, and antioxidants. Blending a small amount into smoothies provides a nutrient boost without overpowering the taste.

- Cauliflower: A versatile vegetable, cauliflower is high in fiber and low in calories. It blends smoothly into smoothies and adds a creamy texture, making it a great alternative to high-calorie thickeners like yogurt or banana.

Sample Recipe Idea

"Green Powerhouse Juice"

Ingredients: Spinach, cucumber, celery, green apple, ginger

Benefits: This juice is hydrating, detoxifying, and packed with antioxidants to support weight loss and overall health.

Section 2: Low-Sugar Fruits

1. Berries for Antioxidants and Fiber

-Blueberries: Rich in antioxidants and fiber, blueberries support brain health, reduce inflammation, and help control blood sugar levels.

- Strawberries: These are high in vitamin C and manganese, aiding in immune health and reducing inflammation. Their sweet, tangy flavor adds brightness to any smoothie.

- Raspberries: Low in calories but high in fiber, raspberries promote digestive health and satiety. They're a great addition to smoothies to add natural sweetness without excessive sugar.

2. Green Apples for Digestive Health

- Benefits of Green Apples: Green apples are lower in sugar compared to other apples and are high in fiber, which supports digestion and keeps you feeling full. They have pectin, a type of fiber that acts as a prebiotic, feeding beneficial gut bacteria.

- Pairing Tips: Green apples add a crisp, tart flavor to juices and smoothies. They work well with leafy greens, celery, and citrus fruits.

3. Citrus Fruits for a Metabolism Boost

- Lemons and Limes: High in vitamin C, these fruits support immune health and help detoxify the liver. Adding a splash of lemon or lime juice to your beverages can enhance flavor while keeping sugar content low.

- Grapefruit: Known for its fat-burning properties, grapefruit helps regulate insulin levels and is high in antioxidants. It's an ideal addition to morning juices for a metabolism boost.

4. Stone Fruits in Moderation

- Peaches and Nectarines: While slightly higher in sugar, stone fruits like peaches and nectarines are nutrient-dense, providing vitamins A and C, fiber, and antioxidants.

- Tips for Use: Add small amounts of stone fruits for flavor variety, especially in summer. Pair them with leafy greens and low-sugar fruits to keep overall sugar content balanced.

Sample Recipe Idea

"Berry Bliss Smoothie"

Ingredients: Blueberries, strawberries, spinach, Greek yogurt, almond milk

Benefits: High in antioxidants, fiber, and protein, this smoothie is perfect for satisfying hunger and reducing cravings.

Section 3: Herbs, Spices, and Superfoods

1. Anti-Inflammatory Herbs and Spices

   - Ginger: Known for its anti-inflammatory and digestive properties, ginger adds a spicy kick to juices and smoothies. It's also known to improve circulation and help with nausea, making it ideal for morning beverages.

- Turmeric: This bright yellow spice has curcumin, a compound with powerful anti-inflammatory and antioxidant effects. Adding a pinch to your smoothie can help reduce inflammation, especially when paired with black pepper for absorption.

2. Metabolism-Boosting Superfoods

- Chia Seeds: Rich in omega-3 fatty acids, fiber, and protein, chia seeds add thickness to smoothies and help keep you full. Their high fiber content promotes digestion and stabilizes blood sugar levels.

- Flaxseeds: These seeds are packed with fiber and lignans, which can improve digestion and support hormonal balance. Flaxseeds also have omega-3s, supporting heart health and weight management.

- Matcha Powder: A concentrated form of green tea, matcha is high in antioxidants and catechins, which may boost metabolism. A teaspoon in a smoothie can add a mild, grassy flavor while enhancing focus and energy.

3. Detoxifying Herbs

- Parsley and Cilantro: Both herbs are rich in antioxidants and chlorophyll, which help detoxify the body. They support kidney function, reduce bloating, and add a fresh, earthy flavor to green juices.

- Mint: Mint is soothing for digestion and pairs well with both fruits and vegetables in smoothies. It adds a refreshing element to drinks and may help curb cravings.

4. Protein-Rich Superfoods

- Spirulina: This blue-green algae are rich in protein, vitamins, and antioxidants. Spirulina can help control appetite and improve energy levels, making it a great addition to any weight-loss smoothie.

- Hemp Seeds: These seeds are high in protein and healthy fats, which support satiety and provide a slight nutty flavor. They're perfect for adding a boost of protein without using dairy or protein powders.

Sample Section: The Benefits of Spices and Superfoods

"Adding ingredients like ginger and turmeric to your beverages can improve digestion and reduce inflammation, aiding in weight loss. Spices not only enhance flavor but also contribute significant health benefits, such as boosting metabolism and supporting detoxification. Superfoods like chia seeds and spirulina are nutrient-dense and help control appetite, making them excellent for long-term weight management."

Sample Recipes and Practical Tips

1. Detox Green Juice

   - Ingredients: Cucumber, celery, parsley, lemon, ginger

   - Benefits: Cleansing and hydrating, this juice supports liver health and digestion, helping to flush out toxins.

2. Turmeric-Ginger Metabolism Smoothie

   - Ingredients: Spinach, green apple, ginger, turmeric, coconut water, black pepper

   - Benefits: Anti-inflammatory and metabolism-boosting, this smoothie is ideal for morning energy.

3. Berry Chia Protein Smoothie

   - Ingredients: Blueberries, raspberries, spinach, chia seeds, Greek yogurt, almond milk

- Benefits: High in fiber, protein, and antioxidants, this smoothie supports satiety and provides sustained energy.

4. Practical Tips for Using Herbs, Spices, and Superfoods

- Use Fresh or Ground Spices: Fresh ginger and turmeric provide the most health benefits, but ground versions are also effective.

- Hydrate Seeds Before Blending: Soaking chia and flaxseeds for a few minutes allows them to expand, improving texture and nutrient absorption.

- Adjust to Taste: Experiment with small amounts to find the flavor balance that works for you, especially with strong spices and superfoods.

Section Summary: Building Nutrient-Dense Beverages

This chapter emphasized the importance of selecting nutrient-packed ingredients to create juices and smoothies that not only aid in weight loss but also support overall health. By incorporating a variety of vegetables, low-sugar fruits, herbs, spices, and superfoods, you can maximize the nutritional value of each beverage and enhance its effectiveness for weight management. From hydrating vegetables and antioxidant-rich berries to metabolism-boosting spices and protein-dense seeds, each ingredient brings unique.

Chapter 3: Meal Planning with Juices and Smoothies

In this chapter, we'll explore how to integrate juices and smoothies effectively into your daily routine for sustainable weight loss and improved health. We'll cover practical ways to replace certain meals with these nutrient-rich beverages, offer sample meal plans for a balanced diet, and provide tips for maintaining this lifestyle long-term. A structured meal plan that incorporates juices and smoothies can help you reach your health goals by ensuring consistent energy, balanced nutrition, and weight management.

Section 1: Incorporating Juices and Smoothies into Your Daily Routine

1. Replacing Meals with Juices and Smoothies

   - Breakfast Replacement: Starting the day with a nutrient-dense smoothie or juice can provide sustained energy and help control cravings. Morning smoothies can include a balance of protein, healthy fats, and low-sugar fruits for satiety and focus.

- Lunch or Dinner Replacement: Using smoothies or juices for lunch or dinner is convenient for busy schedules and helps keep a lighter intake in the evening. Smoothies with greens, a source of protein, and a small amount of fruit can satisfy hunger and prevent overeating.

- Intermittent Fasting with Smoothies and Juices: Juices can be incorporated as part of an intermittent fasting plan, providing nutrients and hydration without breaking a fast. opt for low-calorie green juices in the morning to support fasting benefits.

2. Using Juices and Smoothies as Snacks

- Between Meals: Replacing processed snacks with a juice or smoothie helps prevent energy crashes and provides vitamins and minerals instead of empty calories. Choose options that are high in fiber and protein for lasting fullness.

   - Post-Workout: Smoothies are ideal post-workout snacks that help replenish nutrients, support muscle recovery, and stabilize blood sugar levels. Include protein sources like Greek yogurt or protein powder for best results.

   - Pre-Bedtime Options: For those who feel hungry in the evening, a light smoothie with calming ingredients like chamomile tea, almond milk, and a small amount of banana can promote better sleep.

3. Avoiding Meal Skipping

   - Why Skipping Meals is Counterproductive: Skipping meals can lead to overeating later in the day and disrupt metabolism. Instead, use smoothies or juices as a quick, nutrient-dense choice when time is short.

- **Emergency Smoothie Ideas:** Keep ingredients like frozen berries, leafy greens, and protein powder on hand to quickly blend up a smoothie when you're in a hurry.

4. Proving a Routine

- **Consistency for Success:** Start by replacing one meal a day with a smoothie, then gradually incorporate juices as snacks. Consistency is key to forming healthy habits and seeing results over time.

- **Tracking Progress:** Track your energy levels, weight, and hunger cues to find the right balance. Adjust portions and ingredients based on your body's feedback.

Sample Section

"A well-structured meal plan is essential to maximize the benefits of juices and smoothies. Begin with one smoothie as a meal replacement per day, then gradually add juices in place of snacks for consistent energy and nutrition. By building a routine that includes these nutrient-rich beverages, you'll avoid meal skipping and reduce unhealthy cravings."

Section 2: Sample Meal Plans**

1. One-Week Starter Plan for Weight Loss

   - **Goal: This plan provides a gradual introduction to meal replacements and nutrient-dense snacks with juices and smoothies. It includes one smoothie per day as a meal and a juice as a snack.**

Day	Breakfast	Lunch	Snack	Dinner
Monday	Green Protein Smoothie	Salad with lean protein	Cucumber-Celery Green Juice	Baked vegetables with quinoa
Tuesday	Berry Oat Smoothie	Grilled chicken with veggies	Lemon-Ginger Detox Juice	Vegetable stir-fry with tofu
Wednesday	Avocado-Banana Smoothie	Lentil soup with side salad	Apple-Cucumber Juice	Grilled fish with steamed greens
Thursday	Tropical Spinach Smoothie	Turkey and veggie wrap	Green Apple-Kale Juice	Roasted veggies with chickpeas
Friday	Strawberry-Chia	Veggie-loaded bowl	Beet-Carrot	Stuffed bell peppers

	Smoothie	with hummus	Juice	with rice
Saturday	Matcha Protein Smoothie	Quinoa salad with avocado	Watermelon Mint Juice	Zucchini noodles with marinara
Sunday	Blueberry Almond Smoothie	Mixed veggie stir-fry	Pineapple-Celery Juice	Sweet potato and black bean taco

- **Tips for Success: Prepare smoothies the night before for a quick breakfast and make juices in batches to save time during the week. Adjust part sizes based on your hunger levels and goals.**

2. 30-Day Balanced Meal Plan

- **Goal: A month-long plan to transition into a balanced lifestyle with regular juice and smoothie meals. Each week has a detox day, followed by balanced nutrition on other days.**

- **Detox Days: Once a week, use juices throughout the day to give your digestive system a break while** keeping hydration and nutrients high. Example of a detox day:

- Morning: Lemon-Celery Juice
- Mid-morning: Green Apple-Cucumber Juice
- Lunch: Beet-Spinach Juice
- Afternoon: Ginger-Carrot Juice
- Dinner: Smoothie with kale, cucumber, and chia seeds for gentle satiety

- Regular Days: Combine smoothies and juices as meal replacements or snacks. Aim to have a green smoothie for breakfast and a fruit-based smoothie post-workout or in the afternoon.

3. Sample Day from the 30-Day Plan

- Breakfast: Spinach-Avocado Smoothie (with spinach, avocado, almond milk, chia seeds, and blueberries)

- Lunch: Salad with greens, grilled chicken, chickpeas, and olive oil dressing

- Snack: Ginger-Turmeric Juice (carrot, ginger, turmeric, and a dash of black pepper)

- Dinner: Vegetable soup with lentils and a side of roasted sweet potatoes

Practical Tips for Meal Planning Success

- Batch Preparation: Set aside time to chop and portion fruits and vegetables in advance. Freeze ingredients for smoothies to save time.

- Bottling and Storage: Store juices in airtight containers for freshness and to preserve nutrients. Keep juices refrigerated and consume within 24-48 hours.

- Part Control: For weight loss, ensure smoothies and juices are portioned correctly. Aim for balanced calories with protein, healthy fats, and fiber.

Section 3: Tips for Long-Term Success

1. Finding a Routine that Works for You

- Adapting to Your Lifestyle: Adjust the timing and frequency of smoothies and juices based on your daily schedule and energy needs.

- Adjusting Over Time: As you reach weight-loss goals or enter maintenance, incorporate smoothies and juices in a way that supports long-term health.

2. Setting Realistic Goals

- Start Small: Begin with achievable goals, like one smoothie or juice per day. As you build confidence, increase the frequency or replace more meals if desired.

   - Tracking Progress and Staying Motivated: Keep a journal of your progress, noting energy levels, weight changes, and overall well-being. This will help you stay motivated and make informed adjustments to your plan.

3. Balancing Juices and Smoothies with Whole Foods

   - Integrating Whole Foods: While juices and smoothies are nutrient-dense, whole foods add variety and texture to your diet. Combine smoothies and juices with whole-food meals, such as salads or lean proteins.

   - Listening to Your Body: Pay attention to your body's cues. If you feel overly hungry, add more protein or fiber to your smoothies. Adjust portions to match your activity level and hunger.

4. Adapting the Plan for Social Events and Travel

   - Preparation for Travel: Many juices and smoothies can be prepped in advance or found at juice bars. Look for options with low sugar and fresh ingredients.

   - Staying Flexible: Remember that occasional indulgences are normal and part of a sustainable lifestyle. Return to your routine without guilt and continue making positive choices.

5. Managing Plateaus and Maintaining Motivation

   - Reassessing Your Goals: If progress stalls, consider changing your ingredients or adding more movement to your routine.

   - Celebrate Small Wins: Recognize improvements in energy, sleep, and health as part of your success, not just the number on the scale.

Sample Section

"For long-term success, find a rhythm that fits naturally with your lifestyle. This might mean one smoothie per day, or rotating juices in as snacks and detox options. Setting realistic goals and tracking progress will help you stay motivated, and over time, you'll notice the lasting benefits of integrating these nutrient-packed beverages into your daily life."

Sample Recipe Ideas

1. Morning Green Smoothie

   - Ingredients**: Spinach, cucumber, avocado, chia seeds, unsweetened almond milk

   - Benefits: High in fiber, vitamins, and healthy fats for a satisfying breakfast

2. Citrus Energizer Juice

   - Ingredients: Orange, lemon, ginger, cucumber

   - Benefits: Boosts metabolism and immune function, ideal for morning or midday

Chapter 4: Tailored Juices and Smoothies for Specific Goals

In this chapter, we'll dive into the art of crafting juices and smoothies that target specific health and wellness goals. From fat-burning and detoxification to metabolism-boosting and satiation, each section will provide detailed recipes and ingredient breakdowns designed to maximize benefits in each area. These tailored recipes offer more than just great taste; they're carefully designed to address unique nutritional needs and enhance your weight-loss journey.

Section 1: Fat-Burning Recipes

1. Understanding Fat-Burning Ingredients

- Green Tea: High in catechins, green tea is known to stimulate thermogenesis, helping the body burn fat more effectively. Green tea can be used as a liquid base in smoothies for an added fat-burning boost.

- Cayenne Pepper: The compound capsaicin in cayenne pepper boosts metabolism and can increase the rate at which the body burns calories. Just a pinch adds warmth and a spicy kick to any drink.

- Grapefruit: Known for its ability to lower insulin levels and suppress appetite, grapefruit is a great addition to fat-burning smoothies and juices.

2. Sample Fat-Burning Recipes

- Green Tea Fat Burner Smoothie

  - Ingredients: Brewed green tea (chilled), spinach, cucumber, avocado, chia seeds

  - Benefits: High in antioxidants and fiber, this smoothie helps control hunger and boosts metabolism.

  - Instructions: Blend all ingredients until smooth. Serve at once.

- Cayenne Citrus Fat-Burning Juice

  - Ingredients: Grapefruit, orange, lemon, cayenne pepper, a small piece of ginger

  - Benefits: The combination of citrus fruits and cayenne promotes fat burning and reduces inflammation.

- Instructions: Juice all ingredients and add a pinch of cayenne. Stir well and enjoy.

3. Why These Ingredients Help Burn Fat

- Thermogenesis and Satiety: Ingredients like green tea and cayenne encourage the body to use more energy for digestion, increasing calorie burn. High-fiber ingredients like spinach and chia seeds create fullness, reducing the need for extra calories.

Sample Section

"For a fat-burning boost, try a morning smoothie that includes green tea, spinach, and chia seeds. This combination supports metabolism and provides fiber to keep you full until your next meal."

Section 2: Detoxification

1. The Importance of Detox Ingredients

- Liver-Supporting Ingredients: Ingredients like beetroot, lemon, and turmeric help support liver function, aiding in the body's natural detoxification process.

- Kidney-Supporting Ingredients: Cucumber and watermelon are diuretic, helping the kidneys filter waste and reduce bloating.

- Chlorophyll-Rich Greens: Spinach, kale, and parsley are high in chlorophyll, which helps cleanse the blood and drop toxins.

2. Sample Detox Recipes

- Liver Cleanse Juice

- Ingredients: Beetroot, carrot, celery, lemon, turmeric

- Benefits: This juice is high in antioxidants and vitamins that help the liver process toxins.

- Instructions: Juice all ingredients, stir, and serve. For added benefits, add a pinch of black pepper to enhance turmeric absorption.

- Kidney Flush Juice

- Ingredients: Cucumber, watermelon, mint, lime

- Benefits: Hydrating and refreshing, this juice helps flush out toxins and reduces water retention.

- Instructions: Juice all ingredients and add fresh mint leaves for flavor. Serve chilled.

3. How Detox Ingredients Work

- Antioxidant and Anti-Inflammatory Effects: Beets and turmeric help reduce inflammation and oxidative stress in the liver, supporting detoxification.

- Hydration and Diuretic Properties: Ingredients like

cucumber and watermelon increase urine production, which helps the kidneys remove waste from the body.

Section 3: Metabolism-Boosting Recipes

1. The Science of Metabolism-Boosting Ingredients

   - Green Tea and Matcha: Both green tea and matcha have caffeine and catechins, which can enhance fat oxidation and calorie burn. Matcha, as a concentrated form of green tea, is especially powerful for boosting metabolism.

   - Ginger and Cinnamon: These warming spices increase body temperature slightly, causing the body to burn more calories in response.

   - Apple Cider Vinegar: Known to help control blood sugar levels and suppress appetite, apple cider vinegar is a great addition to metabolism-boosting juices.

2. Sample Metabolism-Boosting Recipes

- Matcha Energy Smoothie
    - Ingredients: Matcha powder, almond milk, banana, spinach, ginger
    - Benefits: This smoothie provides a metabolism boost and sustained energy, ideal for morning or pre-workout.
    - Instructions: Blend all ingredients until smooth and serve at once.

  - Spicy Apple Cider Juice
    - Ingredients: Apple cider vinegar, green apple, lemon, ginger, a dash of cinnamon
    - Benefits: With apple cider vinegar and warming spices, this

juice supports metabolism and digestion.

   - Instructions: Juice the green apple and lemon, then stir in apple cider vinegar, ginger, and cinnamon. Mix well and enjoy.

3. Why These Ingredients Boost Metabolism

   - Thermogenic and Appetite-Suppressing Properties: Ginger, matcha, and apple cider vinegar are known to boost calorie burn and reduce hunger, aiding weight loss and metabolic health.

Section 4: Satiating Smoothies

1. Ingredients for Long-Lasting Satiety

   - Protein Sources: Greek yogurt, protein powder, and nuts add protein to smoothies, which helps control hunger and support muscle maintenance.

   - **Fiber-Rich Ingredients:** Fiber from ingredients like oats, flaxseeds, and chia seeds slows digestion, keeping you full longer.

   - **Healthy Fats:** Avocado, almond butter, and coconut oil are rich in fats that promote satiety and provide a creamy texture to smoothies.

2. Sample Satiating Smoothie Recipes

   - **Protein Power Smoothie**

   - **Ingredients:** Greek yogurt, almond butter, chia seeds, spinach, berries

   - **Benefits:** High in protein and healthy fats, this smoothie keeps you full and provides steady energy.

   - **Instructions:** Blend all ingredients until smooth and enjoy as a meal replacement.

- Fiber-Filled Green Smoothie

   - Ingredients: Avocado, spinach, cucumber, flaxseeds, a splash of coconut water

   - Benefits: Packed with fiber and healthy fats, this smoothie is perfect for keeping hunger at bay.

   - Instructions: Blend all ingredients until smooth. This smoothie can replace breakfast or lunch.

3. How Satiating Ingredients Curb Cravings

   - Protein and Fiber for Fullness: Protein and fiber both slow down digestions, creating a sense of fullness and reducing the urge to snack between meals.

Sample Section

"Adding ingredients like avocado, Greek yogurt, and flaxseeds to your smoothies can help you stay satisfied for hours. The combination of healthy fats, protein, and fiber makes these smoothies ideal meal replacements or snacks for curbing cravings."

Practical Tips for Making Purposeful Juices and Smoothies

1. Timing for Maximum Benefits

- Fat-Burning Smoothies: Best consumed in the morning to kickstart metabolism and provide energy for the day.

- Detox Juices: Ideal during the evening or on an empty stomach to allow your body to focus on detoxification.

- Metabolism-Boosting Drinks: Consume before workouts or in the afternoon to enhance energy and calorie burn.

- **Satiating Smoothies:** Great for meal replacement, particularly for breakfast or lunch to prevent overeating later in the day.

2. Customizing Based on Goals

- **Personalize Ingredient Choices:** Adjust ingredients based on your individual goals. For example, add more greens and fiber if focusing on detox or reduce fruit for lower sugar intake in fat-burning recipes.

- **Experiment with Flavors:** Balance strong flavors (like matcha or apple cider vinegar) with naturally sweet fruits or add spices for warmth without added calories.

3. Storing and Preparing Ahead

- **Batch Prep for Busy Days:** Make ingredients ahead of time by portioning and freezing them. This makes morning smoothies and juices quick and convenient.

- Storing Juices: Fresh juices are best consumed at once, but they can be stored in airtight containers for up to 24 hours. Add lemon juice to slow oxidation and keep freshness.

4. Keeping Track of Progress and Adjusting Recipes

- Monitoring Results: Keep a journal of how you feel after each type of juice or smoothie. Note any changes in energy, hunger, or cravings.

- Adjust as Needed: Based on your body's response, change recipes by adding more protein, fiber, or fat for better satiety or adjusting flavors for enjoyment.

Section Summary: Crafting Juices and Smoothies for Specific Goals

This chapter offered an array of tailored recipes for specific wellness goals, from fat burning and detoxification to metabolism-boosting and satiating drinks. By understanding the unique benefits of various ingredients and combining them strategically, you can create beverages that go beyond basic nutrition and address targeted health needs. These customized drinks offer practical, tasty solutions for weight management, digestive health, and

Chapter 5: Practical Recipes for Weight Loss

In this chapter, we'll dive into practical recipes that support weight loss at each mealtime. From energizing breakfast smoothies to filling midday options and light, digestion-friendly beverages for the evening, these recipes are designed to fit seamlessly into your day. Each recipe is crafted with ingredients that not only support weight loss but also enhance energy, boost metabolism, and provide balanced nutrition. With simple instructions and minimal preparation, these smoothies and juices can easily become part of your daily routine.

Section 1: Breakfast Boosters

1. The Importance of a Nutrient-Dense Breakfast

- Breakfast sets the metabolic tone for the day. Starting with a smoothie or juice that includes fiber, protein, and antioxidants can provide steady energy, reduce cravings, and support metabolism.

2. Key Ingredients for Breakfast Smoothies and Juices

- Green Vegetables: Spinach, kale, and parsley provide fiber and antioxidants without many calories.

- Low-Sugar Fruits: Green apples, berries, and citrus fruits add natural sweetness and are rich in vitamins.

- Healthy Fats and Protein: Ingredients like chia seeds, Greek yogurt, and almond butter add protein and healthy fats to keep you full until lunch.

3. Sample Breakfast Recipes

- Green Energizer Smoothie
- Ingredients**: Spinach, half a green apple, parsley, chia seeds, water or unsweetened almond milk
- Benefits: High in fiber and antioxidants, this smoothie provides energy and helps with digestion.
- Instructions: Blend all ingredients until smooth. Serve immediately.
- Sample Section: "Start your day with the Green Energizer smoothie: blend spinach, half a green apple, a

handful of parsley, and a teaspoon of chia seeds. This combination is packed with fiber and antioxidants, setting a healthy tone for the rest of your day."

- Berry Protein Power Smoothie

   - Ingredients: Mixed berries, Greek yogurt, almond butter, spinach, water

   - Benefits: This smoothie provides protein, antioxidants, and healthy fats, keeping you full and energized.

   - Instructions: Blend all ingredients until smooth. Enjoy as a filling breakfast choice.

- Citrus Kickstart Juice

   - Ingredients: Orange, lemon, ginger, carrot

   - Benefits: Refreshing and rich in vitamin C, this juice is perfect for an immune-boosting start to the day.

- Instructions: Juice all ingredients and serve chilled.

4. Why Breakfast Smoothies and Juices Work for Weight Loss

- Metabolism Boosting: Nutrient-dense breakfasts kickstart metabolism, reducing hunger later in the day.

- Hydration and Detox: Ingredients like cucumber and citrus help hydrate and cleanse the body.

Section 2: Midday Meals

1. Crafting a Filling Midday Smoothie or Juice

- Balanced Macronutrients: Midday smoothies and juices should have a balance of carbs, protein, and fats to satisfy hunger and provide energy for the rest of the day.

- **High-Fiber Ingredients:** Fiber is essential for satiety, helping reduce afternoon cravings and supporting digestion.

2. Key Ingredients for Midday Smoothies and Juices

- **Fiber-Rich Vegetables and Fruits:** Use leafy greens, cucumber, and low-sugar fruits like berries to keep calories low but nutrients high.

- **Protein and Healthy Fats:** Greek yogurt, avocado, and hemp seeds are excellent sources of protein and fats for a more satisfying meal.

3. Sample Midday Meal Recipes

- **Avocado Green Smoothie**
- **Ingredients:** Spinach, avocado, cucumber, hemp seeds, lemon juice, unsweetened almond milk
- **Benefits:** Packed with fiber, protein, and healthy fats, this

smoothie is perfect for a filling lunch.

   - Instructions: Blend all ingredients until smooth. This smoothie is ideal for keeping hunger at bay during the afternoon.

   - Tropical Protein Smoothie

   - Ingredients: Frozen pineapple, mango, spinach, protein powder, coconut water

   - Benefits: This smoothie provides tropical flavors, hydration, and a protein boost.

   - Instructions: Blend all ingredients until smooth. Perfect for a refreshing, nutrient-dense lunch.

   - Super Green Juice

   - Ingredients: Kale, celery, cucumber, green apple, lemon

   - Benefits: Detoxifying and hydrating, this juice is light but full of vitamins and minerals.

- Instructions: Juice all ingredients and serve at once.

4. Why Midday Smoothies and Juices Help with Weight Loss

- Sustained Energy: A balanced midday smoothie can prevent afternoon energy crashes, reducing the temptation for unhealthy snacks.

- Controlled Caloric Intake: Smoothies and juices can replace higher-calorie meals, supporting a calorie deficit for weight loss.

Section 3: Evening Light Options

1. Benefits of a Light, Low-Calorie Evening Beverage

- Evening drinks should be easy on the digestive system and low in calories. These smoothies and juices help satisfy hunger without overloading calories before bed.

2. Key Ingredients for Evening Smoothies and Juices

   - Low-Calorie, Fiber-Rich Vegetables: Cucumber, celery, and zucchini provide bulk without many calories.

   - Relaxing Ingredients: Chamomile tea, almond milk, and small amounts of banana can promote relaxation and improve sleep quality.

   - Digestive Aids: Ginger, peppermint, and fennel support digestion and reduce bloating, making them ideal for evening recipes.

3. Sample Evening Recipes

   - Chamomile and Banana Smoothie

- Ingredients: Brewed chamomile tea (cooled), banana, almond milk, a pinch of cinnamon
- Benefits: This smoothie promotes relaxation and aids digestion before bed.
- Instructions: Blend all ingredients until smooth. Enjoy as a calming evening treat.

- Cucumber Mint Cooler
- Ingredients: Cucumber, mint leaves, lime juice, water
- Benefits: Hydrating and light, this juice helps with digestion and provides a refreshing flavor.
- Instruction: Juice cucumber and mix with fresh mint leaves and lime juice. Serve chilled.

- Ginger Turmeric Digestive Juice
- Ingredients: Carrot, celery, ginger, turmeric, apple cider vinegar

- Benefits: Anti-inflammatory and soothing for digestion, this juice is perfect for the evening.

   - Instructions: Juice all ingredients, stir in apple cider vinegar, and enjoy.

4. Why Light Evening Options Aid Weight Loss

   - Improved Digestion: Low-calorie, fiber-rich evening options prevent bloating and support a good night's sleep.

   - Calorie Control: Choosing a light smoothie or juice in the evening helps keep daily caloric intake balanced and prevents late-night snacking.

Practical Tips for Making and Storing Smoothies and Juices

1. Meal Prep for Busy Mornings

- Frozen Ingredients: Part and freeze ingredients like spinach, berries, and chopped fruits in individual bags to save time in the morning.

  - **Pre-Brewed Teas: Brew green tea, chamomile tea, or other teas in advance and store in the fridge for use in smoothies.

2. Storing and Serving Tips**

  - Freshness: Store smoothies in an airtight container in the fridge for up to 24 hours, but juices are best consumed fresh.

  - Layering for Smoothness: For the best texture, add liquids to the blender first, then softer ingredients, and finally frozen fruits or ice.

3. Part Control and Customization

  - Adjusting Ingredients Based on Goals: For weight loss, reduce higher-calorie ingredients like bananas and avocados, and focus on greens and low-sugar fruits.

   - Experimenting with Flavors: Add a pinch of spices like cinnamon or a few fresh herbs like mint or basil for extra flavor without added calories.

Section Summary: Making Smoothies and Juices Work for Your Daily Schedule

This chapter provided practical, weight-loss-focused recipes for breakfast, lunch, and evening meals, designed to fit various nutritional needs throughout the day. Breakfast boosters provide the energy and nutrients needed to start the day, while filling midday meals sustain energy and prevent cravings. In the evening, light, digestion-friendly options help reduce caloric intake while promoting restful sleep. With these tailored recipes and tips for preparation, you can enjoy smoothies and juices that support your weight-loss goals and fit into any lifestyle.

Chapter 6: Tips and Techniques for Delicious Juices and Smoothies

Creating smoothies and juices that are not only nutritious but also delicious is key to sustaining a healthy lifestyle. This chapter will cover essential tips for enhancing the flavor of your smoothies and juices, balancing ingredients to achieve a perfect taste profile, and best practices for prepping and storing your creations. By mastering these techniques, you'll make every juice and smoothie a delightful experience that you look forward to each day.

Section 1: Improving Taste

1. Natural Sweeteners for Enhanced Flavor

   - Using Fruits to Sweeten Naturally: Low-sugar fruits like berries, green apples, and citrus can add a hint of sweetness without spiking blood sugar.

     - Example: Adding a few strawberries or blueberries can sweeten a smoothie without overpowering it.

   - Adding Creaminess with Banana or Avocado**: For a creamier, naturally sweet flavor, try adding half a banana or a few slices of avocado. Both contribute a subtle sweetness while keeping the texture smooth.

   - Sample Section: "To naturally sweeten your smoothie without adding extra sugar, try adding half a banana or a few berries. Herbs like mint or basil can also add fresh notes that make a huge difference in flavor."

2. Herbs and Spices for Extra Flavor Dimensions

   - Mint and Basil: These herbs add freshness and a cooling effect, especially good for green smoothies or citrus-based juices.

   - Ginger and Turmeric: For a warming, spicy undertone, add fresh ginger or turmeric. Not only do they enhance flavor, but they also provide anti-inflammatory benefits.

   - Cinnamon and Nutmeg: These spices add warmth and depth, pairing well with fruit-based smoothies, especially those having apples or bananas.

3. Natural Flavor Enhancers

   - Coconut Water: Swap out plain water for coconut water to add a hint of natural sweetness and extra electrolytes.

   - Unsweetened Nut Milks: Almond milk, coconut milk, or oat milk can add a creamy texture and mild nutty taste, enhancing the overall experience without added sugars.

   - Vanilla Extract: A small splash of pure vanilla extract can add warmth and subtle sweetness, pairing especially well with berries, bananas, and greens.

Section 2: Combining Ingredients for Balance

1. Balancing Sweet and Sour Flavors

   - Adding Citrus for Tartness: Lemon, lime, and grapefruit add a refreshing tang and balance out the sweetness from fruits. A little citrus goes a long way in cutting through richness and adding brightness to the drink.

- **Pairing Sweet Fruits with Greens:** Sweet fruits like pineapple, mango, and berries pair well with bitter greens such as kale or arugula, creating a balanced taste.

    - **Example:** A pineapple-spinach smoothie balances sweetness with an earthy flavor, creating a delicious contrast.

2. Controlling Bitterness in Green Smoothies

- **Blending with Mild Greens:** Start with mild greens like spinach or romaine, as they're less bitter than kale or dandelion greens. Gradually increase the number of bitter greens as you get accustomed to the taste.

    - **Using Citrus or Sweet Fruits:** Adding orange, mango, or even a bit of apple juice can neutralize bitter flavors.

    - **Balancing with Healthy Fats:** Ingredients like avocado or a tablespoon of almond butter can mellow the bitterness of greens, making the flavor smoother and more enjoyable.

3. Achieving a Creamy Texture

- **Adding Avocado or Banana:** These ingredients provide a creamy texture and natural sweetness. They work well in both fruit-based and green smoothies.

- **Using Greek Yogurt or Silken Tofu:** For a protein boost and creaminess without the sugar, blend in Greek yogurt or silken tofu. Both add thickness and balance to smoothies.

- **Nut Butters and Seeds:** Almond butter, peanut butter, or chia seeds can add creaminess and thickness, making smoothies feel more like a meal.

4. Enhancing Smoothies with Umami and Savory Flavors

- Green Smoothies with Fresh Herb: Fresh parsley or cilantro can add a savory, earthy taste that pairs well with green smoothies.

- Adding a Pinch of Salt: A small pinch of salt can enhance sweetness and bring out the flavors of other ingredients, especially in fruit-based smoothies.

5. Sample Recipe for Balanced Flavors

- Balanced Berry-Green Smoothie
- Ingredients: Spinach, mixed berries, banana, almond butter, almond milk, a dash of cinnamon
- Instructions: Blend until smooth. The sweetness from the berries and banana balances the mild bitterness of the spinach, while almond butter adds a creamy texture and slight nuttiness.

Section 3: Storage and Freshness

1. Best Practices for Preparing Smoothies and Juices in Advance

- Prepping Ingredient: Wash, chop, and portion out ingredients ahead of time. You can store these in the fridge for up to two days or freeze them in individual bags for easy access.

- Freezing Ingredients: Freezing fruits like berries, bananas, and greens helps keep freshness and makes smoothies cold and refreshing. Frozen ingredients also reduce the need for ice, which can dilute flavors.

- Pre-Made Smoothie Packs: Part smoothie ingredients into freezer bags for quick preparation. Just add liquid and blend when ready.

2. Tips for Storing Smoothies and Juices

-Airtight Containers: Store smoothies and juices in airtight containers to reduce oxidation, which can affect taste and nutrient quality. Mason jars with tight lids work well.

- Consume Within 24 Hours: Smoothies are best consumed at once, but they can be stored for up to 24 hours in the refrigerator. Shake well before drinking to redistribute any settled ingredients.

-Adding Lemon Juice to Prevent Oxidation: A splash of lemon juice can help preserve color and prevent browning, especially in smoothies with apples or bananas.

3. Keeping Smoothies Cold and Fresh On-the-Go

- Use Insulated Bottles: If you're taking a smoothie on the go, use an insulated bottle to keep it cool and fresh for several hours.

- Adding Frozen Ingredients Before Storing: If you're storing smoothies in advance, add frozen ingredients to help keep them cold without diluting the flavor.

- Packing Juices with Ice Packs: When traveling with juice, pack it with an ice pack to keep freshness and prevent spoilage.

4. Making Smoothies Last Longer

- Blend Just Before Drinking: For best freshness, blend smoothies right before drinking. If you're short of time, blend the night before and store in the fridge.

- Layering for Longer Freshness: When storing smoothies, add greens or other ingredients that tend to oxidize quickly (like avocado) last to keep the freshness intact longer.

Sample Recipes and Techniques for Flavor Balance and Freshness

1. Minty Green Detox Smoothie

   - Ingredients: Spinach, cucumber, green apple, mint leaves, lemon, water

   - Benefits: Refreshing and detoxifying, with a fresh minty taste that balances the greens.

   - Instructions: Blend all ingredients until smooth. Adding mint and lemon makes this green smoothie light and refreshing.

2. Creamy Tropical Smoothie

   - Ingredients: Frozen mango, banana, coconut milk, a splash of orange juice, and a dash of cinnamon

   - Benefits: This smoothie is creamy and sweet with tropical flavors, balanced by a hint of cinnamon for warmth.

   - Instructions: Blend until smooth and serve at once. The frozen mango adds thickness, and coconut milk enhances creaminess.

3. Cucumber Lime Refresher Juice

- Ingredients: Cucumber, lime, celery, a few fresh mint leaves

- Benefits: This juice is hydrating and has a refreshing tartness from the lime, perfect for hot days or a post-workout drink.

- Instructions: Juice all ingredients and serve over ice. This drink stays fresh for up to 24 hours if refrigerated.

4. Protein Berry Bliss Smoothie

- Ingredients: Mixed berries, Greek yogurt, a handful of spinach, almond butter, almond milk

- Benefits: High in protein and fiber, this smoothie balances tart berries with creamy Greek yogurt and nutty almond butter.

- Instructions: Blend all ingredients until smooth. Berries and yogurt keep it balanced and filling, ideal for breakfast or lunch.

Section Summary: Perfecting the Taste and Freshness of Juices and Smoothies

In this chapter, we explored various techniques to improve the taste, texture, and freshness of your smoothies and juices. By incorporating natural sweeteners like fruits, enhancing flavor with herbs and spices, and balancing ingredients for a harmonious profile, you can create beverages that are both delicious and nutritious. Learning how to store and prep ingredients effectively allows you to keep your smoothies and juices fresh, ensuring that they keep their flavors and nutritional value. Mastering these techniques will make it easy to integrate these healthy, flavorful drinks into your daily routine and enjoy them to their best.

Chapter 7: Developing Healthy Habits and a Mindful Approach to Eating

To achieve lasting success with weight loss and overall health, it's essential to develop healthy habits and practice mindfulness around eating. This chapter will guide you through building consistent, sustainable routines that support long-term wellness. We'll also explore how mindful eating can enhance your relationship with food, helping you focus on satisfaction and enjoyment rather than restriction. Finally, we'll address common challenges, such as cravings, portion control, and staying motivated, providing strategies to help you stay on track.

Section 1: Creating Consistency in Your Routine

1. The Importance of Consistency for Long-Term Success

- Consistency is the foundation of healthy habits. When you repeat positive actions daily, they become automatic, making it easier to support a balanced diet without constant effort.

- Instead of viewing each meal as an opportunity for perfection, aim for gradual, sustainable improvements. Focus on integrating juices and smoothies into your daily routine as simple steps towards health.

2. Building Small, Sustainable Habits

- Start with One Smoothie or Juice Daily: Begin by making one smoothie or juice a day a non-negotiable part of your routine, perhaps as breakfast or an afternoon snack. This small habit can yield significant benefits over time and serve as a consistent nutrient boost.

- **Prove a Set Time for Preparation: Dedicate a specific** time each day for preparing your juices and smoothies, whether it's first thing in the morning or as part of your evening routine. Having a set time makes the habit easier to follow and reduces decision fatigue.

- **Use Visual Reminders and Track Progress: Keep visual reminders,** such as a daily checklist or a visible blender on the counter, to reinforce your routine. Tracking your progress in a journal or app can also help you stay motivated and see how far you've come.

3. Turning Routine into Ritual

- **Transforming your smoothie and** juice routine into a ritual can add enjoyment to the process. Treat this time as a few minutes dedicated to self-care. Play calming music, choose fresh ingredients, and focus on the colors, textures, and smells as you prepare each drink.

   - When you enjoy and look forward to this ritual, it becomes a positive habit that feels like a reward rather than a chore.

Sample Section

"Consistency in your smoothie and juice routine can be a powerful driver for lasting health benefits. Start by integrating just one smoothie or juice into your day, setting up it as a non-negotiable ritual. Dedicate a specific time each day for preparation and enjoy this time as a few moments to invest in yourself."

Section 2: Mindful Eating Practices

1. What is Mindful Eating?

- Mindful eating involves being fully present during meals, focusing on the sensory experiences of food, and tuning into your body's hunger and satiety signals.

- This practice encourages appreciation of each ingredient and can enhance satisfaction, leading to a more balanced and fulfilling eating experience.

2. Practicing Mindfulness with Juices and Smoothies

- Savoring Each Sip: When you drink a smoothie or juice, take the time to notice its color, texture, and flavors. Try sipping slowly, allowing each taste to register, rather than rushing through the experience.

- Paying Attention to Ingredients: Think about the ingredients you're using and how they benefit your body. For example, remind yourself of the antioxidants in berries or the hydration from cucumber. This awareness fosters a positive mindset and gratitude for nourishing your body.

3. Focusing on Satisfaction Rather than Restriction

   - Instead of focusing on what you're "not allowed" to have, approach each meal as an opportunity to nourish and care for yourself. Shifting your mindset from restriction to satisfaction can reduce feelings of deprivation and promote a healthier relationship with food.

   - Recognize the signals of satisfaction and fullness. Stop when you feel comfortably full and savor the flavors and textures of your food rather than overloading your plate.

4. Engaging the Senses for a More Enjoyable Experience

   - Sight, smell, taste, and even sound can enhance your experience with food. Notice the colors of the ingredients, the smell as you blend, and the creamy texture of a smoothie. Being fully engaged allows you to connect with your food, making the experience more satisfying and enjoyable.

Sample Section

"Mindful eating is about being present with your food choices. Enjoy the process of creating and savoring your smoothies, paying attention to the flavors, textures, and benefits of each ingredient. This approach not only enhances the taste experience but also fosters a positive relationship with food."

Section 3: Overcoming Common Challenges

1. Addressing Cravings

- Finding Emotional vs. Physical Hunger: Cravings are often triggered by emotional rather than physical hunger. Before reaching for a snack, pause and ask yourself if you're truly hungry or if you're eating out of stress, boredom, or habit.

- Healthy Substitutes for Cravings: Use smoothies and juices as healthy alternatives for typical cravings. For example:

- Sweet Cravings: Blend frozen berries with a handful of spinach, almond milk, and a dash of vanilla.

- Salty Cravings: Try a green smoothie with celery, cucumber, and a pinch of sea salt, which can help satisfy salty cravings in a nutritious way.

- Distracting Techniques: When a craving hits, try to distract yourself with a 5-10-minute activity, like a short walk, stretching, or deep breathing. Often, cravings will subside when the immediate emotion passes.

2. Managing Portion Control

   - Serving Sizes for Smoothies and Juices: Pre-portion ingredients for smoothies to prevent overeating. A typical smoothie serving is 8-12 ounces, which provides a satisfying snack or meal without excessive calories.

   - Listening to Fullness Cues: Mindful eating can help you recognize when you're full, preventing you from finishing a smoothie or juice out of habit. Start with smaller portions and stop drinking once you feel satisfied.

   - Avoiding High-Calorie Additions: Nut butters, protein powders, and certain fruits can add extra calories. Use measured amounts of high-calorie ingredients and prioritize low-sugar, fiber-rich choices like greens and berries.

3. Staying Motivated

 - Set Small, Achievable Goals: Rather than aiming for drastic changes, set small, specific goals, such as replacing one snack with a smoothie every day. Achieving these small goals will build confidence and motivation.

 - Celebrate Progress: Recognize and reward yourself for staying consistent. Progress isn't just measured by weight loss; celebrate improvements in energy, mood, and overall well-being.

 - Visual Reminders: Keep visible reminders of your goals around the house or at work. A note on the fridge, a recipe book on the counter, or a chart of your daily intake can help reinforce positive habits.

4. Coping with Setbacks

 - Embrace Flexibility: Remember that occasional deviations from your plan are normal and don't signify failure. Focus on getting back on track the next day rather than feeling guilty.

   - Positive Self-Talk: When you meet setbacks, replace negative thoughts with positive affirmations. Remind yourself that each day is an opportunity to continue making positive choices.

   - Seeking Support: Share your goals and challenges with friends, family, or a support group. Talking with others can provide encouragement and accountability, helping you stay focused and motivated.

Sample Section

"Managing cravings and portion control can be challenging, but with mindful strategies, you can navigate these obstacles. For example, if a craving for sweets arises, substitute it with a berry-based smoothie, focusing on natural flavors. Remember, small, consistent efforts add up over time, so celebrate each step toward your goals."

Conclusion: Embracing a Healthy, Mindful Lifestyle

Incorporating juices and smoothies into your diet can go beyond mere weight loss. It's about embracing a healthier, more balanced way of living that center on nourishing your body and enjoying the process. By creating consistent habits, practicing mindfulness, and overcoming challenges with a positive mindset, you're setting yourself up for long-term success and a sustainable approach to health.

- Long-Term Success: Healthy eating is a journey, and there will be highs and lows. Focus on progress, not perfection, and celebrate the positive changes you see in your energy levels, mood, and body.

- Mindful Living: The principles of mindfulness can extend beyond the kitchen. Approach all areas of life with intention, whether it's exercise, rest, or relationships.

- Positive Relationship with Food: Viewing food as a source of nourishment and joy rather than a restriction creates a healthier, more enjoyable approach to eating.

With these practices, you'll find that a healthy lifestyle isn't about strict rules but rather about building a flexible, mindful routine that you enjoy. Embrace each step of the journey and be patient with yourself. A mindful approach to eating can foster long-lasting habits that promote health, happiness, and well-being.

Chapter 8: Keeping Results

Achieving your weight-loss goals is an accomplishment, but supporting those results is where long-term health and wellness are truly set up. In this chapter, we'll explore the steps to transition from a weight-loss-focused diet to a sustainable maintenance plan. We'll cover how to balance juices and smoothies with regular meals, make adjustments for seasonal ingredients and personal preferences, and continue benefiting from the nutritional richness of these drinks. By building a balanced approach, you can keep the weight off and enjoy a varied, satisfying diet for the long run.

Section 1: Transitioning from Weight Loss to Maintenance

1. Understanding the Transition Phase

   - Transitioning to maintenance requires a gradual shift to avoid sudden changes that might cause weight to regain. Instead of stopping your smoothie and juice routine abruptly, make small adjustments to integrate more solid meals over time.

   - Embrace this phase as an opportunity to refine you're eating habits, maintain the nutrition from smoothies and juices, and create a more flexible eating plan.

2. Adjusting Caloric Intake

   - As you transition, consider gradually increasing your daily caloric intake to support a stable weight. Increase portions of whole foods, such as vegetables, lean proteins, and healthy fats, while keeping a nutrient-rich diet.

- If you're unsure about the right caloric level for maintenance, track your meals for a week or two to gauge your needs and adjust as necessary.

3. Reintroducing Solid Foods Gradually

- **Replace One Smoothie with a Whole Meal:** Start by replacing one smoothie with a solid meal that includes a balance of protein, carbs, and fats, such as a quinoa salad with mixed vegetables and lean protein. Continue with one juice or smoothie daily to keep the benefits of nutrient-dense ingredients.

- **Add Whole Ingredients to Smoothies:** For a gradual shift, blend solid ingredients like oats, nuts, or seeds directly into your smoothies. This can help your body adjust to more filling, fiber-rich meals.

- **Incorporate Snacks with High-Fiber Foods:** Add snacks like apple slices with almond butter or a handful of nuts to increase fiber and protein intake throughout the day.

Sample Section

"As you reach your weight loss goals, start to reintroduce more solid foods while keeping a smoothie or juice as part of your daily routine. This will help you maintain the benefits of nutrient-dense drinks while expanding your dietary variety and enjoying more satisfying meals."

Section 2: Balancing Juices and Smoothies with Regular Meals

1. Keeping the Benefits of Smoothies and Juices

- Even in maintenance, smoothies and juices offer a quick, easy way to consume essential vitamins, minerals, and antioxidants. They can also serve as convenient options for busy mornings or post-workout recovery.

- Continue to use these drinks as an added source of fruits, vegetables, and superfoods to complement a well-rounded diet without relying on them exclusively.

2. Creating a Balanced Daily Routine

- Use Smoothies as Snacks: Incorporate smaller smoothies as snacks between meals, with a focus on lower-calorie, fiber-rich ingredients to prevent overeating.

- Morning Smoothie Routine: Start your day with a smoothie packed with greens, low-sugar fruits, and protein. This keeps breakfast light yet nourishing, setting a positive tone for the rest of the day.

- Juices for Nutrient Boosts: Use juices, especially green juices, as nutrient boosts when you feel your vegetable intake is low. They're great for hydration and can easily be added as an afternoon refresher.

3. Integrating Solid Meals with Nutrient Density

- **Focus on High-Protein, High-Fiber Meals:** Balanced meals that include lean protein, fiber, and healthy fats are filling and support metabolic health. Aim for meals like vegetable stir-fry with grilled chicken or roasted salmon with quinoa and greens.

- **Healthy Carbohydrates:** Include whole grains, sweet potatoes, and legumes to support sustained energy levels, especially if your activity level has increased since weight loss.

- **Colorful Vegetables:** Keep a variety of colorful vegetables on your plate to keep the antioxidant and vitamin benefits of your juicing days.

4. Sample Meal Plan for Maintenance

   - Breakfast: Green smoothie with spinach, cucumber, banana, chia seeds, and unsweetened almond milk.

   - Lunch: Grilled chicken breast with mixed greens, cherry tomatoes, quinoa, and avocado.

   - Afternoon Snack: Carrot and ginger juice or a handful of almonds with an apple.

   - Dinner: Baked salmon with roasted sweet potatoes, steamed broccoli, and a side salad with olive oil dressing.

Section 3: Adapting to Different Seasons and Preferences

1. Seasonal Ingredient Swaps

   - Spring and Summer: Use fresh, light ingredients like cucumber, watermelon, berries, and leafy greens for refreshing smoothies and juices.

  - Fall and Winter Swap in seasonal produce such as pumpkin, apples, pears, and root vegetables like carrots and beets. Warm spices like cinnamon and ginger add comfort and seasonal flavor.

  - Year-Round Staples: Keep some staple ingredients like spinach, frozen berries, and bananas available throughout the year to ensure you have a variety of flavors and nutrients.

2. Keeping Your Diet Exciting with New Recipes

  - Try new smoothie and juice recipes that match the season or explore new ingredients you may not have used before, like persimmons in fall or tropical fruits like mango in summer.

- Rotate superfoods like spirulina, chia seeds, or flaxseeds to enhance variety and nutritional benefits without changing your routine drastically.

3. Adjusting Recipes for Warmer or Cooler Drinks

- Cooler Weather: opt for room-temperature smoothies or warm ingredients like oats or spices. Try blending in brewed chamomile or ginger tea for warmth.

- Warmer Weather: Keep it cool with frozen ingredients like berries, coconut water, and a few ice cubes. Mint, basil, and citrus can add refreshing notes to any drink.

4. Sample Seasonal Recipes**

- Spring Detox Smoothie: Spinach, cucumber, green apple, mint, lemon, and water.

- Summer Tropical Juice: Pineapple, mango, coconut water, and lime.

- Fall Spice Smoothie: Pumpkin puree, almond milk, a banana, cinnamon, and a dash of nutmeg.

- Winter Warm-Up Juice: Carrot, orange, ginger, turmeric, and a splash of apple juice.

Section 4: Keeping Motivation and Balance

1. Setting New Health Goals Beyond Weight Loss

- Maintenance is a time to focus on holistic health rather than just the scale. Consider goals like improving energy levels, enhancing mental clarity, or building muscle.

- Create a flexible plan that includes physical activity, self-care, and balanced eating. For example, challenge yourself to try a new type of workout or experiment with cooking healthy meals at home.

2. Tracking Progress Without Focusing Solely on Weight

   - Instead of focusing exclusively on weight, consider other metrics such as waist circumference, energy levels, sleep quality, and overall mood.

   - Use a health journal to track your meals, how they make you feel, and other wellness indicators. This can help you find patterns and adjust as needed.

3. Supporting Mindful Eating Practices

   - Continue the mindful eating habits you developed during weight loss. Enjoy your meals without distractions and listen to your body's hunger and fullness cues.

   - Remember to savor each bite and appreciate the flavors,

textures, and nutritional benefits of each meal. This approach helps prevent overeating and keeps you connected to your body's needs.

4. Celebrating Milestones and Staying Flexible

- Celebrate small victories, like supporting your weight, trying new foods, or successfully making healthier food choices over time.

- Flexibility is key to sustainability. Allow yourself to enjoy occasional indulgences without guilt. Balance is essential and letting yourself enjoy your favorite treats in moderation helps you stick with healthy habits for the long term.

5. Sample Section

"Maintaining motivation after weight loss means shifting your focus from numbers on the scale to overall wellness. Set new goals, like improving your fitness or energy levels, and continue tracking progress in ways that matter to you, such as enhanced mood or better sleep."

Conclusion: Building a Lasting, Balanced Approach to Health

Transitioning from weight loss to maintenance is about finding balance and creating a routine that fits your lifestyle and long-term goals. By gradually introducing more solid foods, balancing juices and smoothies with whole meals, and adapting your diet to seasonal changes, you can enjoy a varied, satisfying approach to healthy eating. Keeping motivation high through new goals and mindful eating practices will help you sustain your progress and celebrate the positive effects of a well-balanced lifestyle.

- **Sustainable Health Over Quick Fixes:** Maintenance is a lifelong journey, and consistency is more valuable than perfection. Focus on daily habits that support your well-being and fit naturally into your life.

- **Embracing Flexibility:** Allow for changes as your lifestyle, preferences, and health goals evolve. Maintenance isn't static; it's about adapting and enjoying the journey.

- **The Role of Juices and Smoothies in Long-Term Health:** Even in maintenance, juices and smoothies can provide a quick, effective way to meet your nutritional needs. Use them as complements to a balanced diet rather than relying on them exclusively.

With this approach, you'll find that maintenance is not only achievable but also enjoyable, as you nourish your body, mind, and lifestyle with flexibility and balance.

Lose Weight without Diets and Drugs (Easy, Healthy, Simple)

This book offers a refreshing approach to weight loss, replacing restrictive diets with the nourishing power of juices and smoothies. Perfect for those looking for a sustainable, enjoyable way to shed pounds, boost energy, and enhance well-being, it turns nutrient-rich drinks into effective tools for a healthier lifestyle.

Beginning with the benefits of juices and smoothies, the book highlights how these drinks make weight loss simple and satisfying. You'll learn to balance proteins, fats, and carbs,

incorporate fruits, vegetables, and superfoods for optimal results, and follow easy meal plans that fit seamlessly into daily life. With recipes tailored for detox, fat-burning, and metabolism-boosting, the variety ensures you'll stay on track with ease and flavor.

Key chapters include:

- The Basics of Juices and Smoothies for Weight Loss: Understanding the unique benefits and uses of each.

- Healthy Ingredients and Their Properties: Low-sugar fruits, leafy greens, and superfoods for powerful results.

- **Diet and Nutrition Plan: Weekly and monthly guides for detox, accelerated weight loss, and long-term balance.

- Practical Recipes for Weight Loss:

Morning, midday, and evening options to fuel your day.

- **Tips and Techniques:** Flavor-enhancing advice for delicious, fresh drinks.

Beyond recipes, the book offers insights into developing lasting habits, practicing mindful eating, and transitioning to maintenance without losing results. It encourages viewing food as nourishment and enjoyment, helping you build a balanced, sustainable lifestyle.

Whether your goal is to lose weight, improve health, or add variety to your diet, "Lose Weight without Diets and Drugs" is a guide to achieving it with ease, flavor, and satisfaction. Embrace this path to wellness with juices and smoothies and discover how delicious healthy living can be!